T013316?

ONE OUT OF EVERY 16 AMERICANS WILL GET COLON CANCER. If colon cancer is found early, then most people live. If colon cancer is found late, then only 5% of people will live.

You've been scheduled for a colonoscopy. **Colonoscopy can find cancer and can save lives.** This booklet will help you get ready. We know it can be challenging to get ready for a colonoscopy. We also know that you may have many questions about the test. We created this booklet to help answer your questions. After you read this booklet, go to page 17 and **complete the checklist** as you prepare for your procedure.

This booklet was developed by talking to people who had a colonoscopy. Researchers asked these people to explain what was confusing or difficult about getting ready for the test. The researchers then used the feedback to create this booklet, and then tested the booklet in a study to see if it could help people get ready for the colonoscopy. The study found that people who read the booklet were more likely to have a clean prep compared to those who did not get the booklet.*

About Getting Ready

The MOST IMPORTANT thing you can do is to **empty out your colon by carefully following the diet described in this booklet and taking your "bowel prep" medicine prescribed by your doctor.** We want to help you get ready. If you come in with your colon properly emptied out, then we can make this "ONE AND DONE." **"One and done" means just that: let's do this once, do it right, and then be done. Then we won't run the risk and inconvenience of asking you to come back and repeat the test.**

* Spiegel BM, Talley J, Alvarez E, Bolus R, Kurzbard N, Ho A, Kaneshiro M, Cohen H. Impact of a novel patient educational booklet on colonoscopy preparation quality: results of a randomized controlled trial. Gastroenterology 2010;A387 (Digestive Disease Week, New Orleans, LA)

How does a colonoscopy work?

The purpose of a colonoscopy is to look inside your large intestine (colon) for polyps, cancers, ulcers, and other conditions. Just before the procedure starts, you will receive some medicine to make you sleepy. Most people do not remember having the procedure. The doctor will pass a flexible tube as shown below. The tube has a small camera and a headlight which allow the doctor to see the inside of your colon on a TV monitor. The doctor can take biopsies of abnormal areas, and can also remove polyps. You will wake up shortly after the test is over.

Colonoscopy examines the entire length of the colon; **sigmoidoscopy** examines only the lower third

Here is a picture of how it works. The scope bends as it passes through the colon. The headlight provides light so the doctor can see. The scope is passed through the whole colon. It goes farther than a sigmoidoscopy, which only looks at part of the colon.

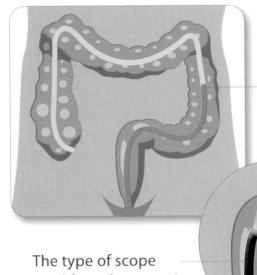

End of sigmoidoscopy

Small headlight so the doctor can see

The type of scope used for colonoscopies

Why is it Important to Get Clean on the Inside?

Your doctor **must** be able to see in order to do the test right. If it is dirty on the inside, then your doctor may not see important things, like polyps or cancer, and may even have to do the test again. That would mean you would have to start over, and nobody wants to do that. So help us help you to make this "one and done."

Imagine This:

Think of it this way: a clean colon is like driving on a country road on a sunny day. A dirty colon is like driving in a snowstorm.

When your colon is clean, doing the colonoscopy is like driving on a country road on a sunny day. It's easy to see and easy to drive.

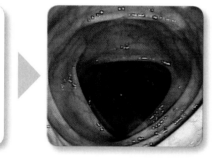 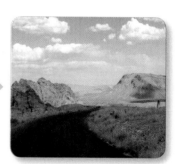

When your colon is dirty, doing the colonoscopy is like driving on a winter road in a snow storm. It is hard to see and hard to drive.

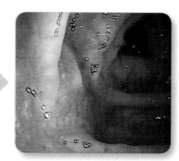 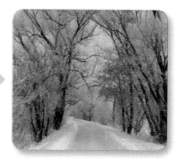

ONE DAY Before Your Colonoscopy

What you Eat

You must not eat any solid foods the day before your colonoscopy. You may only eat a clear liquid diet. Go to page 8 for things you can eat.

What you Drink

You must drink only clear liquids for breakfast, lunch, and dinner. Be sure to drink at least 12 tall glasses (at least 8-10 ounces each) of clear liquids throughout the day in addition to what is instructed for your bowel prep.

Taking your "Prep"

By the day before your test you should already have your "bowel prep" medicine. If not, call your doctor. The instructions for your prep are located inside the prep box. **You will start taking your prep at 6:00 pm the evening before your test.** Follow the directions carefully. How do you know if your prep is working? Go to page 13 to find out.

Some doctors want you to take the whole prep the night before your test. But many doctors prescribe a "split prep." A "split prep" means you will take half of the prep the evening before the test, and the other half the day of the test. Check the instructions from your doctor. **If your doctor prescribed a "split prep," then you will take the first part of your prep at 6:00 pm the evening before your test, and you will take the second part of the prep the morning of your test starting 4 hours before the scheduled time of your colonoscopy.**

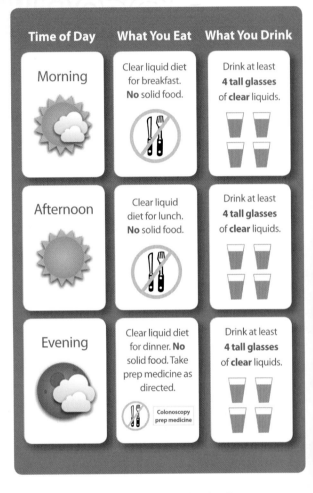

Time of Day	What You Eat	What You Drink
Morning	Clear liquid diet for breakfast. **No** solid food.	Drink at least **4 tall glasses** of **clear** liquids.
Afternoon	Clear liquid diet for lunch. **No** solid food.	Drink at least **4 tall glasses** of **clear** liquids.
Evening	Clear liquid diet for dinner. **No** solid food. Take prep medicine as directed. Colonoscopy prep medicine	Drink at least **4 tall glasses** of **clear** liquids.

What you Eat

You must not eat any solid foods prior to your colonoscopy, even if your colonoscopy is scheduled for the afternoon. You can eat a regular diet once you are fully awake after the test is over.

What you Drink

You must drink only clear liquids prior to your colonoscopy. Be sure to drink at least 2 tall glasses (at least 8-10 ounces each) of clear sports drink with electrolytes prior to your colonoscopy.

Taking Your Prep

If your doctor ordered a "split prep," then you must take the **second part** of your prep the morning of your test. Be sure to take it 4 hours before your test, even if that means having to get up very early. For example, if your doctor prescribed a "split prep" and your test is scheduled for 1:00 pm, then take the second part of your prep at 9:00 am the morning of your test. If your procedure is earlier in the morning, then this means you will have to get up very early to take this second part of your prep. We know it is hard to get up this early, but

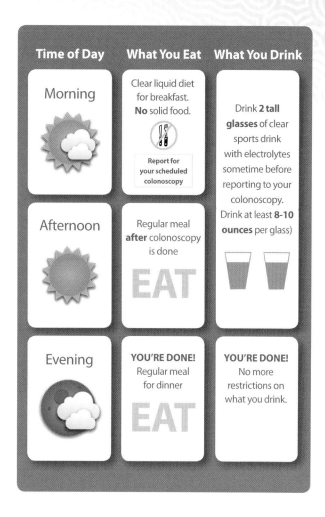

Time of Day	What You Eat	What You Drink
Morning	Clear liquid diet for breakfast. **No** solid food. Report for your scheduled colonoscopy	Drink **2 tall glasses** of clear sports drink with electrolytes sometime before reporting to your colonoscopy. Drink at least **8-10 ounces** per glass)
Afternoon	Regular meal **after** colonoscopy is done EAT	
Evening	YOU'RE DONE! Regular meal for dinner EAT	YOU'RE DONE! No more restrictions on what you drink.

it is very important that you take the second part of your prep 4 hours before your colonoscopy in order for the prep to work.

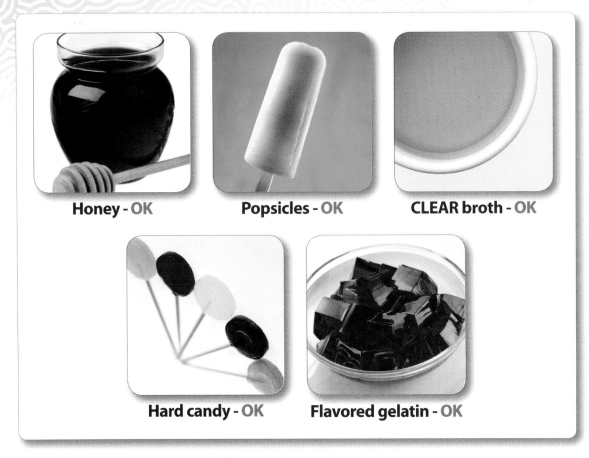

Honey - OK

Popsicles - OK

CLEAR broth - OK

Hard candy - OK

Flavored gelatin - OK

What about Red Food?

You may have heard that red food is not acceptable when
preparing for a colonoscopy. However, there are no studies to
show that red food makes any difference to the success of your
procedure. When people follow all the instructions in this booklet
they usually end up with clean preps, even if they eat red foods.
But some doctors prefer that their patients avoid red foods; if so,
your doctor should let you know about this restriction.

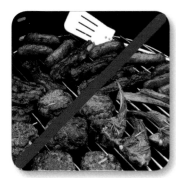

No meats - **NOT OK**

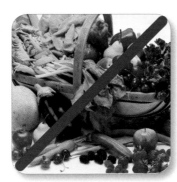

No vegetables - **NOT OK**

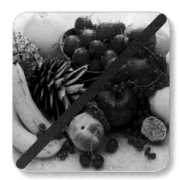

No fruits - **NOT OK**

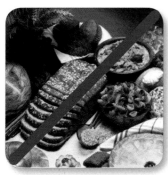

No breads, grains, rice, cereals - **NOT OK**

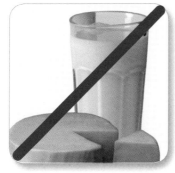

No milk and dairy products - **NOT OK**

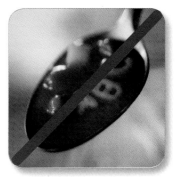

No soups with vegetables, noodles, rice, meat or other chunks of food - **NOT OK**

What Drinks Are OK?

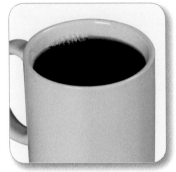

BLACK coffee - OK

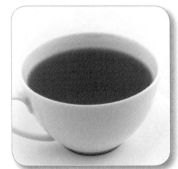

Tea - OK

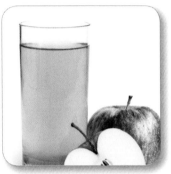

Apple juice - OK

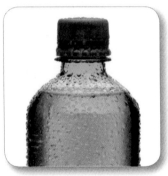

Soda pop, ginger ale, and club soda - OK

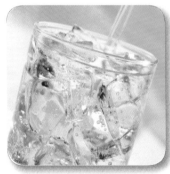

Water and mineral water - OK

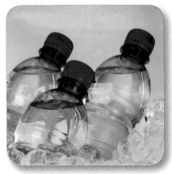

CLEAR sports drink with electrolytes - OK

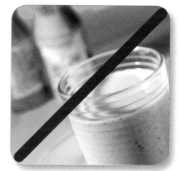

No milk - NOT OK

No milkshakes - NOT OK

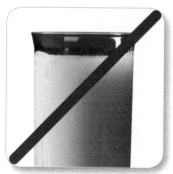

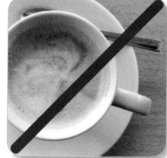

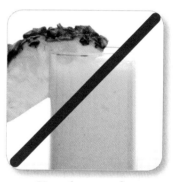

No orange juice - NOT OK

No coffee with cream - NOT OK

No pineapple juice - NOT OK

What about Alcohol?

Although alcohol is a clear fluid, it can make you dehydrated. You should NOT drink alcohol during the preparation for your test.

What is a "Clear Liquid"?

As you get ready for your colonoscopy, you must only drink clear liquids. A liquid is "clear" if you can read something through it. Use this simple test to figure out what you can drink, and what you cannot drink.

This is orange juice. It's not clear, because you can't read newspaper print through it. **Don't drink this.**

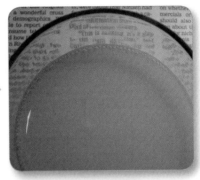

This is pineapple juice. It's also not clear. **Don't drink this.**

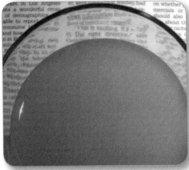

This is apple juice. You can read newspaper print right through it. **You can drink this.**

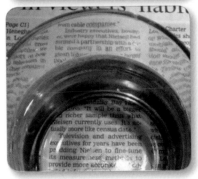

How do You Know When Your Prep is Working?

The stool coming out should look like the stuff you are eating and drinking – clear and **without many particles.** You know you're done when the stool coming out is **yellow, light, liquid, and clear** – like urine. Below is a guide to help.

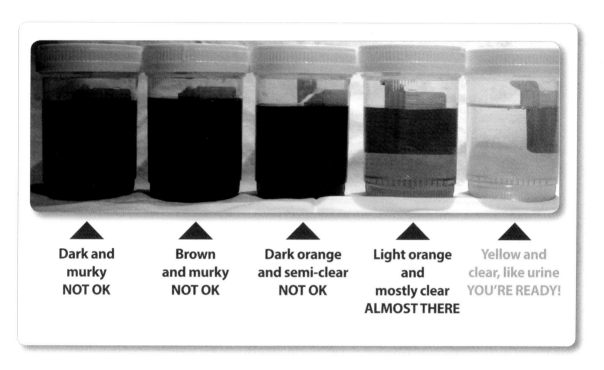

| Dark and murky NOT OK | Brown and murky NOT OK | Dark orange and semi-clear NOT OK | Light orange and mostly clear ALMOST THERE | Yellow and clear, like urine YOU'RE READY! |

Frequently Asked Questions

Can I drive myself home after my colonoscopy?

NO. You will receive medication to make you sleepy during the test. That means you cannot drive home. You must arrange for someone to drive you home after the test. You may use public transportation (taxi or bus), but only if you have an adult who can escort you home.

How long will the test take?

The test itself usually takes 10-30 minutes. But expect to spend the entire morning and part of the afternoon at the Medical Center to have the test and to recover from any sleeping medicine. If you arrive between 6:30 AM and 7:00 AM, you likely will be ready to go home by late morning or very early afternoon. If you arrive later, you may not be ready to go home before very late afternoon. Call your doctor if you have any questions about the timing of your colonoscopy.

What if I take blood pressure medicines?

If you take blood pressure medicine, be sure to still use the medicine while preparing for the test. On the day of your test, you should take your blood pressure medicine with water at least 2 hours before your test. Be sure to call your doctor if you have any questions about how best to take your blood pressure medicines prior to the test.

What if I take aspirin, clopidogrel, or Plavix®?

Some people need to stay on these medicines even if they are going to have a colonoscopy. Other people should stop taking these medicines before their colonoscopy. Please check with your doctor to find out whether you should, or should not, continue taking these medicines prior to your colonoscopy. If your doctor says it is okay to stop, then plan to stop taking these medicines one week before your colonoscopy. You will continue these medicines after the test, unless otherwise instructed by your doctor.

What if I take an anti-inflammatory medicine, like Motrin®, Aleve®, Ibuprofen, Naprosyn®, or Naproxen?
Depending on the specifics of your procedure, it may be okay to continue taking these medicines. But check with your doctor for more information.

What if I take a blood thinner like Coumadin® or warfarin?
You may have already received instructions on how to take your Coumadin® or warfarin prior to the colonoscopy. If not, then please check with your doctor as soon as possible to determine how to proceed. You will continue to take your Coumadin® or warfarin after the colonoscopy unless your doctor gives you other instructions.

What if I take diabetes medicines?
If you are diabetic, take half of your diabetes medicine while on the clear liquid diet. Then, do not take your medicine on the morning of the test. You will resume your medicines after the test. Please check with your doctor if you have any further questions or concerns about these medicines.

My prep hasn't started working yet. Is that OK?
Different people respond differently to the bowel prep—some people start having diarrhea within minutes of taking the prep, while others have no response for an hour or more. If you have waited more than 3 hours without a response, then it may not be working well. Be sure you are drinking enough fluid, as instructed on page 5. If that doesn't work, take the second part of your prep and continue to drink fluids. It should work eventually. Call your doctor if the medicine is still not working at all despite drinking enough fluid and taking the medicine as prescribed.

Frequently Asked Questions

How do I know when my bowel prep is complete?

You know your bowel prep is complete when your stool becomes clear and yellow, as described on page 13. If your stool becomes clear before completion of your prep, please continue taking your full prep as instructed.

What if I take fish oil?

STOP taking fish oil two days before your colonoscopy. You can continue taking this after the test, unless otherwise instructed by your doctor. Please check with your Primary Care Physician if you have any further questions or concerns about these instructions regarding fish oil.

What are the side effects of the "bowel prep"?

You will have lots of diarrhea from the bowel prep. This will start anywhere between a few minutes to 3 hours after you start the prep. You will spend a lot of time on the toilet once you start taking the prep. So plan to be home, and plan to be near a toilet. Most people have bloating and abdominal discomfort. This is normal. Do not be alarmed if you feel these symptoms. Many people have nausea. This is also normal. Some people do not like the taste or smell of the medicine. Please do not let this get in the way of taking the medicine as directed. Rarely, some people throw up while taking the prep. If this happens, stop taking the prep and call your doctor.

Colonoscopy Checklist

Instructions:

Here's a checklist of things to do as you prepare for your colonoscopy.
As you do each one, check it off the list by marking an "X" in each box.
Make sure each box has been checked prior to coming in for your procedure.

Before you Start

- [ ] Read the booklet carefully.
- [ ] Make sure you have your bowel prep kit. If not, call your doctor.

One Day Before your Colonoscopy

- [ ] Eat breakfast – clear liquids only, no solid foods.
- [ ] Eat lunch – clear liquids only, no solid foods.
- [ ] Eat dinner – clear liquids only, no solid foods.
- [ ] Take bowel prep in the evening as instructed.
- [ ] Drink at least 12 tall glasses of clear liquids throughout the day.

Day of your Colonoscopy

- [ ] If your doctor prescribed a "split prep," take the **second part** of bowel prep as instructed, starting 4 hours before your colonoscopy.
- [ ] Drink 2 tall glasses of clear sports drink prior to your appointment.
- [ ] Report for your colonoscopy as instructed.

Notes